Conversations With Myself
Managing the Madness of My Mind

Suzanna Fraire

Copyright © 2023 Suzanna Fraire
All rights reserved. ISBN: 9781916808447
Printed in the United States of America.

No part of this publication shall be reproduced, transmitted, or sold in whole or in part in any form without prior written consent of the author, except as provided by the United States of America copyright law. Any unauthorized usage of the text without express written permission of the publisher is a violation of the author's copyright and is illegal and punishable by law. All trademarks and registered trademarks appearing in this guide are the property of their respective owners.

For permission requests, write to the publisher, addressed "Attention: Permissions Coordinator," at the address below.

Amazon Book Publishing Center 420 Terry Ave N, Seattle, Washington, 98109, U.S.A

The opinions expressed by the Author are not necessarily those held by Amazon Publishing Center.

Ordering Information: Quantity sales and special discounts are available on quantity purchases by corporations, associations, and others. For details, contact the publisher at info@amazonbookpublishingcenter.com.

The information contained within this book is strictly for informational purposes. The material may include information, products, or services by third parties. As such, the Author and Publisher do not assume responsibility or liability for any third-party material or opinions. The publisher is not responsible for websites (or their content) that are not owned by the publisher. Readers are advised to do their own due diligence when it comes to making decisions.

Amazon Publishing Center works with authors, and aspiring authors, who have a story to tell and a brand to build. Do you have a book idea you would like us to consider publishing? Please visit AmazonBookPublishingCenter.com for more information.

This book is dedicated to my children, Jorge, Joe, and Rigo. You have been my deepest love, fiercest strength, and greatest hope. Thank you for loving me through it all.

Special thanks to my dear niece, Valentina. I will always be your biggest fan, amongst others. Thank you for your help and support in allowing this book to go from a dream to a reality. I couldn't have done it without you. And to the Fraire family. I wouldn't be me if it wasn't for you.

Acknowledgements

Thanks for all the support, advice, wisdom, and teachings:
Monica Montoya
Jax Atlantis
Breeonika Dell
Jennifer Gilchrist
Neighbor Don

TABLE OF CONTENTS

Introduction..1

Part 1—My Story..2

CHAPTER 1
Understanding Trauma...18

CHAPTER 2
Unraveling the Impact of Abuse: A Deep Dive into Mental, Emotional, Physical, and Financial Manipulation...24

CHAPTER 3
Ancestral/Cultural Trauma...27

CHAPTER 4
Societal Trauma and Its Impacts..32

CHAPTER 5
DNA, Hereditary Illness, and Trauma: An Unseen Connection................36

CHAPTER 6
Mental Blocks and The Impact of a Closed Mind: Barriers to Growth.....39

CHAPTER 7
Cognitive-Behavioral Therapy (CBT), Dialectical Behavioral Therapy (DBT), Neuro-Linguistic Programming (NLP), Trans Magnetic Stimulation (TMS) and Meditation: Tools for Healing and Growth.............................43

Conclusion..48

Resources...49

Suzanna Fraire

INTRODUCTION

    Imagine losing everything—your marriage, your job, even your will to live—only to realize that the biggest battle you face is not in the world around you but within the corridors of your own mind. Six years ago, this was my reality.

    Over the last six years, after losing my 20+ year marriage, my mom, my job, and almost my life, I have learned the true meaning of resilience. My story is not just about a downward spiral but about the journey I undertook to reclaim myself and the wisdom I have gained along the way. My decisions and actions affected not only me but those around me as well. It changed the course of my life.

    The challenge was not only to recover from my losses and the suicidal despair but also to confront the fears and limitations that had trapped me in my own self-created hell. If I was going to redeem myself in my children's eyes, I had to get my life together. I decided to embark on this journey of self-discovery and lead a purpose-filled life. I was no longer willing or able to white knuckle it. So, I embarked on a journey of self-discovery and transformation, and in this book, I will guide you through the steps I took to free myself from my mental and emotional shackles.

    With this book, it is my hope that through my process, you will uncover the hidden fears and blocks that hold you back from your true potential and learn how to overcome them. I challenge you now to dig deep to find out what you a truly capable of.

    Join me as I recount my journey through managing the madness of my mind. It is my wish that through my journey, you may find a lesson or a sign that guides you on your path to live your life to the fullest. I hope you enjoy the ride!

- In love and light,
  Suzanna Fraire

Conversation With Myself
Managing the Madness of my Mind

PART 1—MY STORY

In the midst of my 21-year marriage ending in divorce, I had just lost my mother, and it felt like the darkness had finally claimed victory. I was exhausted. I had grown tired of shouldering the world's weight, and now, I found myself thrust into the raging fire alone. I was left with big shoes to fill. I certainly didn't feel ready for this enormous task.

The memories of my mother oscillate, varying from day to day. They are intertwined with my moods and influenced by what transpired in my external environment. My mother was the cornerstone of our family. She was my rock. Every person who knew her had a tale to share - some uplifting, others more ominous.

Reflecting upon it, I strongly suspect that my mother may have been grappling with an undiagnosed mental illness, perhaps bipolar disorder, or borderline personality disorder. It seems plausible, given my own diagnosis. Our personalities mirror each other in numerous ways. My mother had a generous spirit, and she gave everything she had to everyone around her. But she was also brutally honest and always managed to call people out on their bullshit.

My mother, Debbie, was not just a rock but the very foundation upon which I built my life. She was a survivor in every sense of the word. Enduring immense physical abuse inflicted by her own father, she soldiered on. She lived through the horrific ordeal of being raped by a classmate, followed by his subsequent murder at her father's hands. Her first marriage was marked by a relentless onslaught of emotional, physical, financial, and mental abuse, yet she thrived.

The death of her mother was a painful blow, yet she endured it. Even as she witnessed her children follow a similar, tumultuous path, she fought to endure as long as she could, always aiming for the greater good. However, in moments when her past trauma overshadowed her present, those who knew her found themselves treading on eggshells.

Her moods were unpredictable, and her words often cut. You never cared who she might offend, and she was not afraid to meet physical justice. Whether it was a man or a woman, adult, or child, if you overstepped boundaries in her eyes, you were about to learn a harsh lesson. Despite her mercurial nature, my mother's struggles are a testament to her strength, resilience, and indomitable spirit. She was, is, and will forever be my guiding force.

Reflecting on my childhood, I've come to comprehend the choices my parents made and the life they strived to provide for us. We resided in a neighborhood known for its infamy, often branded as a hotbed for gang activity. Yet, ironically, my memories of childhood remain overwhelmingly positive and joyous.

My brother, brimming with charisma, embodied loyalty to such an extent that it often became his downfall. Despite the loving and nurturing environment provided by our parents, he found himself ensnared in the pitfalls of gang life at an early age.

Our home was a community hub of sorts. My dad and uncles, joined by neighborhood kids, would play football and baseball in our yard or in the streets. They would fill the truck with eager children and embark on adventures to the roller rink or Great America—this was before Marine World graced Vallejo with its presence. They even formed a softball team that rivaled other families in town and surrounding areas.

My mother, meanwhile, was the nourishing force that sustained us all. Always prepared with snacks to feed an army of kids, her capacity to stretch resources was nothing short of miraculous. We lived a humble life by conventional standards, yet she made it seem as if we had it all. Her secret? A shift in perspective—it wasn't about how things would materialize, but about having the faith it would happen, no matter what.

And make things happen she did. For instance, how did she know the Wonder Bread delivery man would bring his truck loaded with day-old goods, instead of discarding them, to our doorstep? We savored a feast of Twinkies, Ho-Hos, Suzy-Q's, cupcakes, and more. After the kids had their fill, she would meticulously stock the cabinets, planning for the month ahead. With a monthly paycheck, careful planning was a necessity. Or getting 20 nosebleed tickets to the A's games and taking as many neighborhood kids along.

My parents showered us with love and support, with no lack of discipline, setting an example for us to follow. My brother, to the outside world, may appear as a villain; but in my eyes, he is a savior. He taught me that embracing the role of a villain isn't necessarily a bad thing. Every story needs its antagonist, and if one must assume this role, why not strive to be the best? This was our mindset. We understand that we all have roles to play in this grand game of life, and the key to thriving lies in adapting to the ever-changing rules of the game.

    Much like our mother, my brother and I are empaths, absorbing and sharing in the emotions of others so that no one must walk their journey alone. We understand the pain of loneliness and choose to lower our vibrations, allowing others to rise. Yet, we fail to realize that this act of selflessness creates a ripple effect, impeding our personal growth.

    I understand the choices my brother made. I observe his community, the strength of their bond, their loyalty, and their mutual dependence. Their shared pain fosters a bond only they can fully comprehend. "Change your environment before your environment changes you" - this has been an impact on my family. We were a unit, never divided by race, religion, or economic status. We simply existed harmoniously together. I see who he had to become so that others around him, including myself, could thrive. I remember times when these hard-core gang members would come to the house and sit and cry to my mom. She would help them make sense of things. She never turned anyone away, from strangers knocking on our door at 3 AM looking for milk and diapers for their babies to hungry neighbors stopping by just as we were unloading our latest Costco run and then leaving with their bellies full and some snacks for the road. I will never forget the day when a neighbor notorious for showing up and asking for handouts showed up at her door after over 20 years to pay back a loan of a hundred dollars. My mom cried hard that day. She had never expected to see that money again, and she couldn't believe that after all this time, he would make do with his promise to pay her back. It wasn't ever about the money. It was about keeping your word, no matter what.

    My life could have been much worse. My biological father abandoned me before I was born. Yet, he occasionally entered our lives, always leaving a trail of pain and suffering in his wake. My mother, driven by an idealistic hope, believed that preserving a connection between us would somehow nurture a father-child bond and that would eventually lead to healing. But, by permitting him to intermittently disrupt our lives as he pleased, she was perpetuating the cycle of abuse she herself had endured from her own father and later, from him.

It wasn't until she met the man, whom I proudly call my dad, that a significant shift occurred. He taught her that love was not synonymous with suffering and that it should bring joy, not pain. He guided her in establishing and upholding boundaries, opening her eyes to the damage this sperm donor was causing. His narcissistic tendencies were wreaking havoc on our lives. Our biological father was abusive - physically, emotionally, and in my case, sexually. As I matured, I began to understand the profound influence this had on my life. It led to unhealthy relationships with men, a sense of unworthiness, and the perpetual feeling of being sexualized and unseen. I anticipated abandonment, sometimes provoking conflict to expedite the inevitable.

On the flip side, my brother and I were fortunate to have our "real" dad in our lives. He provided us with a sense of balance, unconditional love, and steady support. He also introduced an aspect of healthy discipline that was missing in our lives. My mother, in her misguided way, thought the way to correct us was through harsh physical punishment. I remember waking up to belt lashes for not properly washing the dishes the night before. Random slaps in the face because she was angry at someone else. I think the most humiliating thing for me was the day I tried to wake her up to drive me to school. I was about 13 or 14, I believe. I entered her room to let her know that it was getting late and that if she didn't take me, I would have to leave to catch the bus. She didn't respond. As I go to open the front door to head to the bus stop, she comes storming out, screaming at the top of her lungs. I turned to respond and was met with a hairbrush slap across my face. I was done. I do not know what demon arose inside and instinctively slapped her back open handed. Boy, was that a mistake. I don't even remember blinking when I was on my back bearing the entirety of her 300-pound self, straddling my defenseless body. She was whaling her fists at my face, and the only thing I could do was cover myself with my arms to minimize the damage. All the while, the front door had remained open, and all the neighborhood kids paused for the show as they made their way to the bus stop.

Conversation With Myself
Managing the Madness of my Mind

My dad, however, tried to teach her the virtues of patience and communication. He was one to give exhaustive lectures about why our actions were wrong rather than resorting to physical punishment. I remember begging him for a beating just to get him to shut up. He would talk and still does, for hours upon hours, explaining his points repeatedly. A broken record is an understatement. There were one or two times that he resorted to spanking, and I admit my brother and I deserved it. We were hellions. We fought worse than cats and dogs.

My dad weathered the minor storms like my brother's spontaneous joyride to San Francisco in our father's brand-new pickup truck or the times we ditched school to indulge in teenage mischief. Yet, there was a glaring gender bias. My brother was treated leniently because he was a man, while I was put on house arrest. The patriarchal culture we were part of posited that women should primarily engage in housekeeping and child-rearing while maintaining obedience. My mother defied these stereotypes, yet he loved her, nonetheless. I often felt he was molding me into a milder version of her.

In my teenage years, I encountered a shift in my parents' attitude. This is where the cultural and ancestral traumas come into play. They became overprotective, dictating what I wore and how I behaved within the confines of the family, inhibiting my social interactions under the pretext that "friends don't exist." I grew up wary and mistrustful of others and not fully prepared to navigate the complexities of social interactions. As per cultural norms, I wasn't allowed to date until I was fifteen. When that time came, I was under constant surveillance. I wasn't taught to trust my own instincts and make my own decisions and associate with the people that I felt I needed to grow and evolve. Everyone had to be family approved. I recall attending dances with an entourage of what I felt were bodyguards just so I could meet boys. Potential suitors had to navigate not only my parents but also a defensive line of uncles and cousins. And once they passed that test, they had to contend with my brother.

This daunting gauntlet unintentionally instilled a "princess complex" within me. I held what I thought at the time were high standards for those who wanted to enter my life, and if they failed to meet them, they were quickly dismissed. This mindset led me to believe that I was too demanding or "too much," – which led to my downfall, a perception that took a lifetime to unlearn.

At the age of 19, I met a man who effortlessly surmounted every barrier I'd set. A whirlwind romance followed, culminating in a marriage just seven months after our first encounter. We spent 21 years together in a union that was, in no uncertain terms, challenging. He needed a partner who was nurturing and resilient, someone who would stand in his corner when the world turned against him. As our relationship reached its final stages, I could only envision the strain he must have experienced. We had entered a stage of mutual discomfort, not so delicately tiptoeing on eggshells around each other, inadvertently causing deeper wounds with each passing day.

During our marriage, my ex-husband attempted to manage my emotional instability by adopting various tactics. He would withhold love, affection, and financial support, using them as punishment or reward contingent on my compliance. Our communication suffered, leading to isolation and loneliness that was more severe than actual solitude. The internal voices that proclaimed that I was too much or not enough were continually echoed in his actions. There was a clear lack of compromise on his part when it came to my personal aspirations. He failed to acknowledge me as an individual with independent needs and dreams, constantly craving control. At this point, I had fallen deeper into the confines of our Hispanic culture. A woman is to be seen and not heard. We are to maintain a perfect household, raise proper children, make sure the bills are paid, food is on the table, laundry is done, be everyone's taxi, and still be available for sex on demand. I was pressured into this lifestyle, believing I was doing the right thing, and I was. But I was lacking. I was lacking emotionally, spiritually, and towards the end, financially. I would get frustrated or upset, and he was never my soft spot to fall for. My wants, my needs, and my dreams never mattered. He worked, he made good money, and we were surviving. But I wanted attention, I wanted vacations, I wanted him to show me how proud of me he was by showering me with the things I thought I needed. Why couldn't we live like those around us? Taking family vacations, going camping, running around theme parks, and exploring the world around us, giving our children the luxury of life experiences. Why did it have to be about money all the time? Knowing we had the money but choosing to hoard it instead. Money was a huge factor in our marriage, and the mismanagement of it was our downfall. I realize now that we could have had the perfect marriage had we just communicated properly and compromised. Instead, when he punished me with neglect or harsh words for something that he didn't agree with, I would retaliate and hit him where it hurt his wallet. I developed an unhealthy coping mechanism for addiction. Initially, it was just shopping. Buying anything that gave me a moment of instant gratification. Something, anything really to make me feel good. I started investing in the MLM (multi-level marketing) schemes to feel validated and try to earn a living to afford the things I wanted and needed without asking for permission and still be home with my children. The women in my neighborhood seemed to excel in this. So, I blindly followed their lead. Ending up in massive debt and my ex forcibly having to bail me out time and again was too much for him. He couldn't see that he was hurting me, and I couldn't see that I was hurting him. We were not communicating to understand one another. We communicated to be heard and be right. Never getting to the root of the problem and never creating a plan of action. Never sitting down to compromise and support. And this is why our marriage failed.

At this point, what I desperately sought was self-control - control over my emotions, finances, and the ability to recognize my own worth. Until then, my decisions had been unduly influenced by others. I felt obligated to embody the 'perfect' wife and lover, forcing myself to maintain the household and ensure meals were prepared, even though domesticity was not my forte. My abhorrence for cleaning, not to mention laundry, was evident. I was expected to be perpetually available for my husband's sexual needs. The societal expectations of being the 'perfect' mother added to my stress, with continuous volunteering, over-involvement, and self-sacrifice aimed at proving my worth.

My ex-husband lacked comprehension of personal growth and was resistant to change. His inability to understand my struggles meant he couldn't provide adequate support. I don't blame him for this. I had to navigate my way through the labyrinth of addiction and self-destruction in order to establish a sturdier foundation for myself. This process was the predominant cause for our divorce. I was spiraling out of control, and I refused to drag him down with me any longer. The union had become toxic for us and our families. I could not, nor would not, continue the patterns of an unhealthy relationship.

At this stage, I was morphing into the person I had vowed never to become and had resorted to self-medicating as a coping mechanism. I wanted to erase all the torment, to shove it out of sight and out of mind. However, this approach only led me further down the path of self-destruction. I was feeding the flames of my self-sabotage because I felt unworthy. As a result, I felt the need to push everyone away. I was spiraling, and my family did not deserve to be part of this.

I gave him every reason to despise me because I loathed myself. And it worked; he despises me to this day. He lives with that hatred, but I've now come to understand that I don't need him to love me, hate me, or even comprehend me. I did the best I could, gave all I was capable of giving at the time, and I was a good wife, a good mother – just not in the way he had envisioned. I was who I needed to be in those moments in order to survive. I've come to terms with it now. Oprah said in one of her shows, "When you know better, you do better" This has been my mantra.

He gave me every reason to despise him. But, despite everything, we were what we needed to be for each other at the time, even though, sadly, it wasn't enough. He provided me with a sense of stability and security, always ensuring his family was taken care of financially. In doing so, he isolated himself and turned to vices to manage his responsibilities. The burden of the world seemed to rest on his shoulders, with my added baggage only increasing the load. Not only did he financially support our children and me, but he also took care of his parents and funded his sisters' college education, enabling a change in generational patterns within his family. His parents, distant and set in their ways, lacked the affection and hands-on approach we adopted. He filled those gaps and offered more. His contributions to my life and those around him were truly significant. It is unfortunate that we had no proper means of communication, which ultimately led to our marital demise.

At the time, we were both blind to the bigger picture - how to synergize our strengths and weaknesses to form a robust partnership. We lacked effective communication skills, and he was particularly resistant to acquiring them. Therapy or counseling was never an option due to the machismo of our

Conversation With Myself
Managing the Madness of my Mind

culture. Men don't need help. It was then that I realized I needed to be the catalyst for change. I was worn down, trying to rationalize my feelings, exhausting myself by persistently trying to make him see that life wasn't meant to be this stagnant, monotonous sequence of events. I learned that change, growth, and evolution are inevitable and necessary. I needed to evolve beyond the detrimental cycles and patterns that had characterized my existence for so long. The reality dawned on me: there wasn't a knight in shining armor coming to save me or fix me.

This was about transcending the hurt I had endured all of my life and resolving never to allow myself to feel that way again. This was about me facing my own traumas of sexual abuse as a child at the hands of the man that was "supposed to be my dad" and dealing with helicopter parents, force-feeding me their customs, values, and traumas alike, well into my married years and how that paved the way to failure. This was about acknowledging and taking responsibility for the role I played in my own life – how I let my inner thoughts, feelings, and personal struggles manipulate my behavior and responses. I had to do this myself. Realizing that no one could fix me, but it was a monumental ah-ha moment.

Those who know me well or have encountered some version of me understand my propensity to be candid, sometimes aggressively so. I tend to bottle up my feelings until someone inadvertently triggers an emotional explosion, a barrage of words that may not be the most pleasant or tactful. In many ways, this will always be a part of me - a trait influenced by my Libra tendencies, constantly in search of balance. However, I teeter on the Scorpio cusp, and when balance eludes me, I can sting.

I no longer needed to be this person, perpetually reactive to how others perceive and judge me. I don't want nor need to fight every moment of every day for self-control and a sense of self-worth or constantly defend myself and my actions with an unruly fierceness, trying to get those around me to understand.

For so long, I've been the dependable "go-to" girl, prioritizing the needs of others before addressing my own. I've built my life on the principle of treating others the way I want to be treated. Yet, I was often met with a lack of reciprocation, failing to receive the same level of loyalty, love, and respect that I readily extended. I overextended myself and took on too much, mirroring my mother's approach to life. Yet, I realized that such relationships were unhealthy and unfair. Why couldn't I accept what I deserved? Why did I settle for crumbs when I had the potential and right to own the damn whole bakery?

I had to embark on a profound journey of personal transformation. It required me to alter the narrative I had been living by, to unlearn the beliefs and teachings that no longer served me. I recognized that to truly embrace my authentic self, and I needed to let go of the external influences and expectations that had shaped me. It was a process of rediscovering the person I was born to be and reconnecting with my true essence. I had to replace the addiction of instant gratification with acceptance and self-care.

Setting and maintaining boundaries became a crucial aspect of this transformation. I had to learn what my limits were and have the courage to assert them in various aspects of my life. By doing so, I regained a sense of control and self-respect, enabling me to foster healthier relationships and prioritize my well-being.

As I delved deeper into this journey, I became aware of recurring patterns and behaviors within myself. Recognizing these patterns was instrumental in understanding the root causes of my struggles. It was a profound moment of self-reflection and introspection. This marked the true beginning of my transformational path. Because the question was never, why do these things happen to me? The question always is, what can I learn from this situation? When you start with a learning mindset, the lessons become rewarding, and the trials and tribulations of life become comical adventures.

In my quest for growth and healing, the therapies and methods outlined later in this book played a significant role. The therapeutic approaches of CBT, DBT, and NLP helped me discern my actions and self-talk, providing me with valuable insights into the factors that led me to my present state. At the same time, meditation allowed me to be present in my energy and to physically manifest feelings of joy, abundance, and self-love. CBT taught me to take action and move in the motions of success. DBT specifically shed light on my thoughts, beliefs, and judgments about myself that I had held as unquestionable truths. It prompted me to revisit every painful experience I had endured, the times when I felt hurt, betrayed, violated, unseen, and unheard. Through the lens of an impartial observer, I examined each of these experiences, aiming to understand them from a new perspective.

I acknowledged that many of the things that had happened to me were beyond my control. While I couldn't change the past, I realized that I had the power to determine how I allowed those experiences to impact my present and future. I consciously chose not to carry the weight of those experiences any longer. I no longer wanted to exist in a perpetual state of fight or flight, which had taken a toll on my mental and physical well-being. The multitude of psychological and physical diagnoses had left me feeling numb and detached. Thus, I shifted my focus from merely surviving the trauma to actively overcoming it. I redefined what it meant to heal and grow from those experiences.

Actively changing the voices in my head using the tools in the later part of this book became imperative. Instead of listening to the destructive inner demons that haunted me, I sought guidance from my inner angels—the positive, empowering aspects of myself. This required me to confront a whole new world within, challenging my preconceived notions and expanding my understanding of my own potential.

In this transformative process, the science behind it provided a logical framework for understanding the steps I needed to take. However, I also recognized the importance of tapping into my spiritual senses. Neuro-Linguistic Programming (NLP) emerged as a pivotal tool, teaching me the significance of my internal thoughts and my subsequent trauma responses in the form of my reactions to trigger situations. And with the guidance of meditation as a means of connecting with my inner self, I found solace, clarity, and a deeper connection to my spirituality. I forged a new alliance with my inner self. Searching deep for my true passion and purpose in this life, I reluctantly embarked on this never-ending journey of self-discovery.

By employing these various tools and techniques, I am strategically overcoming the obstacles that have hindered my growth. This isn't a one-click fix. This is a life-long process. I carved out a new path for myself—one that aligns with my authentic self, my aspirations, my values, and my core beliefs and found uncompromisable boundaries that set the stage for the change that I so desperately needed. This transformation not only impacted my own future but also had a ripple effect on those I love. By prioritizing my well-being and personal growth, I became better equipped to contribute positively to the lives of others, fostering stronger, more fulfilling relationships.

My journey of transformation required me to change my narrative, unlearn outdated beliefs, rediscover my true self, establish and uphold boundaries, recognize patterns and behaviors, and overcome the impact of past experiences. The combination of CBT, DBT, and NLP provided me with invaluable insights and tools to navigate this path. It was a holistic approach that merged the logical understanding with the spiritual connection, ultimately enabling me to create a brighter, more fulfilling future for myself and those I hold dear. I am able to understand my thought process and listen to my higher self (i.e. Gut feelings or intuition). And I am able to understand and dominate the aspects of my addictive behaviors.

I had to force myself to relive the processes that created this unwanted version of myself. It is not an easy process, nor should it be, but it is worth it. I had to ask myself why these traumas, limitations and blocks were weighing so heavily on my heart? Why was I allowing my past to dictate my future and my overall happiness? Why was it ok for me to live an unhealthy life? Then I had to take it a step further and start looking at the future that I wanted. What was within my control to change? What steps do I need to take to achieve my goals and dreams of a happy, abundant life? We cannot change or control the things that are not within our power. I had to let go of the fact that these things I felt so horrible about happened to me. I had to travel back in time and change those negative aspects to realize what I could have done differently and act today as if I had. I do not own what others have done to me that I feel have negative impacts on my life. I can only own how I allowed them to control and manipulate my inner voice and reset my own mindset. I had to change the way I felt about each situation.

Now I could go on and on about all the bad things that happened to me in detail, each instance of physical abuse that I endured at the hands of my mother, my bio-dad and my brother, that later trickled into every romantic relationship. I can go into detail about how these men have manipulated me, used me to better themselves or just saw me as a sexual pleasure. But we all have our own experiences with personal details. Our stories are not the same, but the feelings that are left are the same. Loss, abandonment, betrayal, fear, anger, frustration, loneliness, these are just a few. I'm sure the list of feelings is overwhelmingly long for each of us. It is in recognizing that these feelings were never ours to carry with us, but they were necessary to overcome for growth.

Neurolinguistic Programming (NLP) was a watershed moment in my personal growth. Being a highly empathic individual, to the degree of insanity, I can readily absorb the energies of others - an ability that is both overwhelming and awe-inspiring. NLP was the first framework I encountered that merged my lifelong meditation rituals with cutting-edge science. It illuminated the power of directed problem-solving within my meditative practices.

I am a firm believer in the statement that we are born equipped with all the knowledge and innate wisdom we need for this life. This belief guided me in deciphering my mind and establishing a healthier boundary between my personal energy and the energies of the external world. What burdens was I carrying? Were they within my control? What changes could I implement to reset, refocus, and rise above my predicaments? It isn't easy living in a constant state of inquiry, but it led me to a point where I was no longer exploited and started prioritizing my well-being first. NLP showed me how to utilize Cognitive Behavioral Therapy (CBT) and Dialectical Behavior Therapy (DBT) techniques during meditation to dive deep into my psyche for answers. The journey was unsettling and frightening, but I was at rock bottom, my life in disarray, having lost everything I held dear, my marriage, job, financial security, and with my mother's inspiring presence missing from my life, I was lost. With no money, no family, and no true foundation of who I was or where I wanted to be, these tools became a lifeline, a path toward regaining a sense of normalcy.

The role of frequencies in my transformation cannot be overstated. It's known that certain frequencies have healing effects. For instance, 40Hz has demonstrated positive impacts on Alzheimer's and Parkinson's disease. Other frequencies have shown benefits in stroke recovery, reduced pain perception, cancer treatments, and even enhancing Neurogenesis and physical rehabilitation. Human beings have a remarkable ability to perceive a wide range of vibrational frequencies and amplitudes. Thus, making it possible to self-heal. It's an area of ongoing research, but there's evidence that the vibrations and frequencies in our everyday environments significantly influence our overall well-being and mental state. Whether it's the type of music we listen to or the ambiance of our neighborhood - a bustling city or a serene countryside - frequency is everywhere. It sets the tone for our daily lives.

Through frequency and meditation, I noticed the vibrations within my body alter. It was as if I could physically sense my cells transforming. Diving deeper into this phenomenon, I discovered that combining meditation with specific frequencies had a profound effect on the physiology of my body and mind. Coupling this practice with the therapeutic approaches of CBT, DBT, and NLP, I began healing the internal facets of my life, which, in turn, manifested in physical recovery.

People ask me all the time, "How do you meditate? I get monkey mind when I try." My response to that is I allow the monkeys to play. It is during meditation that I tap into my demons and dig deep and ask myself, 'Why is this at the forefront of my mind?' I ask myself, "Why am I allowing myself to be trapped by these memories, feelings, or blocks?" And then, I go deeper and say, "What is one thing that I can do differently each day to get out of this state that I am in and move forward to what I need to focus on, which are my goals and dreams?"

Once crippled by fibromyalgia, rendering me bedridden for weeks due to incessant pain, I regained my mobility, started exercising, and embraced life again. I could experience touch without the reflexive response of pain. I could wake up and stand immediately, a feat previously impossible. My migraines, once a thrice-weekly torment, vanished over two years. My arthritis pain transformed from debilitating to unnoticeable. I was no longer dependent on pain medications or psych meds, for that matter. I made the conscious decision to remove all pharmaceuticals from my life and start managing my mental illness on my own. Now, let me state that I am not opposed to big pharma, nor do I recommend stopping or starting any medications without the proper guidance from professionals. Please understand that all my transformations have been under the strict guidance of a magnificent healthcare team, which consists of a psychiatrist, psychologist, general practitioner, astrologer, psychic advisors, spiritual coaches, friends, and family. These are people that I have chosen to work with that are compatible with my energy and my fundamental beliefs. It is important to recognize who you have in your circle and maintain that energetic balance. We all have the capacity to tap into our higher selves, and each process looks different to each of us. This is why it is so important to focus on our inner selves because as we focus on the external self, we are doomed to live superficial lives without purpose or meaning. Only going through the motions and always wishing for things to be different. Because no matter who you are, what you do, or your financial status, if you are not living in your higher self, you will always lack something. Be it love, loyalty, respect, money, or an array of material possessions, you will always be in search of yourself. Once you find yourself, everything falls into place.

 I began experimenting with myself. Like in the movie LUCY, I needed to experience my brain's capacity. What if I could increase it each day? How far would I get without taking it too far? They say that psychics and intuitive use a higher brain capacity for their ability to see beyond the veil. To seep through the matrix and touch the other side. Some call it manifestation, some call it prayer, some call it magic either way, it exists. It is all just a transfer of energy. We choose to label things to our understanding, not realizing that it's all-inclusive. We have indigenous tribes on separate sides of the world performing similar rituals distinct from their culture. The foundations are fundamentally the same. Religion is just a limitation on fundamental belief systems derived from a human experience. I choose not to limit myself within the confines and beliefs that others impose. I choose to listen and learn and take whatever fits my soul's purpose and carry it with me. The baggage I carry now is filled with a hunger for knowledge and experiences, not the weight of my past. I recognize that who I am now is uncomfortable for those who are not ready or willing to evolve. Like my best friend says, "Not my monkey." I understand that people do not believe in what I do. The only thing that matters is that I am clearing my karma and that of my descendants so that lessons can be learned. It is a never-ending cycle. And I ask if you're reading this book to take a chance and focus on your higher self. What is it that you need? What are your desires? I challenge you to do the hard work now, so your future self or descendants don't have to. I leave you with the words of Tony Robbins, "Weak people create bad times, bad times create strong people, and strong people create great times." This is the cycle of life, and it has proven true for me. Let us together create great times.

PART 2–MY PROCESS

CHAPTER 1 - UNDERSTANDING TRAUMA

Section I: Defining Trauma

Trauma is a deeply distressing or disturbing experience that imprints itself onto our minds. It comes in many forms, just as I experienced during my solo car accident. The terrifying sound of twisting metal, the sight of a 20foot wooden light pole crashing down on my entire vehicle, the thoughts of my infant child in the back seat and terror that consumed me remembering the unborn child I was carrying—these memories linger on, a testament to the traumatic nature of the event.

Trauma can also be the loss of a loved one to a terminal illness or as disturbing as sexual abuse. Trauma comes in various forms. It can be physical, mental/psychological, emotional/verbal, sexual, financial, and even cultural and social. Trauma is whatever hurts us so deeply that it changes who we are at the time and changes who we are supposed to become.

Section II: The Mind's Defense Mechanisms

Anna Freud defined the mind's defense mechanisms as "unconscious resources used by ego" to ultimately decrease internal stress. People often conceive these unconscious mechanisms to reduce conflict within themselves.

Our brains have evolved to prioritize our safety, creating comfort zones and fostering a fear of the unknown. This can often lead us into a state of stagnation, avoiding progress and change as we cling to what we perceive as safe.

This improves our system's response to threats. The amygdala (figure 1) is the part of the brain that activates a person's fight-or-flight response and is responsible for releasing the stress hormones cortisol, catecholamine, and vasopressin. These hormones and their responses are designed to help us deal with stressful situations. For example, encountering a dangerous animal during a walk. Your body reacts to stress and releases the hormones to which we respond through fight, flight, freeze or fawn. Chronic and continuous exposure to stress leaves this portion of the brain in a constant state which has dire effects on our mental and physical health.

An overactive amygdala triggers a person's state of being in constant fear, anger, anxiety, or obedience. Hence the fight, flight, freeze or fawn reactions. Fight =anger; Flight=fear; Freeze=anxiety; Fawn=obedience. These are just examples.

Cortisol increases blood sugar levels, boosting energy production while suppressing digestion, reproduction, and immunity. Constant high levels lead to weight gain and depression, among other things.

Catecholamines are a group of hormones consisting of epinephrine, norepinephrine, and dopamine. These are neurotransmitters that send signals between nerve cells to assist the body's response to stress.

Epinephrine increases heart rate, blood pressure, blood flow and energy boosts to muscles. Excess can lead to anxiety, irritability, and difficulty sleeping.

Norepinephrine is released in smaller amounts and is similar to epinephrine in its effects, with the added effects of hypervigilance and alertness.

Dopamine is the mood hormone that plays a role in motivation and pleasure. It is commonly known as the "reward hormone or happy hormone." Although researchers are still investigating, research states that it is essential for coping with stress as it allows for adaptation to various environmental stimuli, which brings me to my theory of addiction.

Whether it be drugs, alcohol, sex, gambling, etc., it provides an escape.

Vasopressin, an antidiuretic hormone, helps regulate blood pressure and water metabolism. Excess production increases blood pressure and shoots the kidneys into hyper-function, reabsorbing water from urine, which leads to less urine production.

Regulating these hormones decreases health risks, such as heart disease, stroke, depression, anxiety, memory loss, brain fog, cognitive decline, chronic fatigue syndrome, gastrointestinal problems, weakened immune system, weight gain, hair and skin problems, and sleep problems.

As children, we can't control what happens to us, but as adults, we must learn how to react and process situations to make the necessary changes to improve our quality of life and create processes for future generations. For example, a child who has experienced some type of physical abuse and does not then learn to process the situation will be forced to react in accordance with their internal response mechanisms. Which, when left untreated, creates negative patterns and behaviors designated by our own individual response systems. In turn, teaching a child to be mindful opens them to more positive experiences throughout life. Guiding them to make the best choices within their circumstances.

Section III: The Role of Mindset

What is mindset? Mindset is a powerful force in our lives. It is influenced by various factors, including trauma, cultural programming, societal programming, DNA, and mental/physical health. Our thoughts play a crucial role in how we perceive our reality and navigate through it.

The following are things that form a mindset:
- Trauma - physical, mental, emotional and/or financial pain, manipulation and/or suffering endured at any point in life.
- Cultural Programmingrace, religion, ancestry (family), ethnicity, beliefs
- Societal Programming – friends, coworkers, political parties (persons you choose to associate with)
- DNA- hereditary issues
- Mental/Physical Health – your fight/flight/freeze response and the effects it has on our bodies.

These will be covered in depth in Chapter 3.

The role mindset plays in our day to day is simply becoming consciously aware at all times of how we feel in the present moment, why we feel the way we do, what external factors play into the current situation and what we can do to change it. We will go into more detail in Chapter 2.

Section IV: Personal Journey: Confronting the Past

I was thirty-three when I decided to face my past to unlock the suppressed memories from my childhood. As a "fixer" who was always there for others, I often neglected my personal issues. It was as if I was stuck in survival mode due to the childhood trauma that I hadn't fully confronted.

I found my ability to give and receive love was hindered by my childhood experiences of abuse and abandonment. It created trauma responses that often propelled me into toxic situations that I mistook for surface-level issues.

I started therapy but found myself on a rollercoaster ride of diagnoses and medication. The demands of being a mother, a daughter, a wife, and a board member, coupled with my health challenges, left me with little space to prioritize myself.

As I navigated the tumultuous seas of my mind, I was amazed at the brain's capacity for self-healing and suppressing traumatic memories. This led me to question the brain's capabilities and potential further.

During one of my therapy sessions, I unearthed suppressed memories of sexual abuse. These revelations offered insights into my trauma response and its influence on my behavior. I began to understand that part of healing involved forgiveness and self-awareness.

Section V: The Power of Confronting Trauma

Our society often encourages us to suppress our emotions to avoid confronting our pain. Yet, leaving trauma unaddressed only leads to further

Conversation With Myself
Managing the Madness of my Mind

complications. I have learned that it is important to face our "demons," to understand them and to learn from them. It is important to recognize within us and teach our children the things (be it situations, places, people, behaviors etc.) that do not align with who we are, are not acceptable. Focusing on our higher purpose because we are all created for a purpose. Creating and maintaining boundaries are essential to self-preservation.

My journey has led me to reflect on the various forms of trauma and their profound impact on personal development. As I look back, I realize that we have the power to choose how we respond to our trauma. It is my hope that my story will encourage others to confront their past and embark on their own journey of self-discovery.

In this book, I pledge to guide you through an intimate understanding of trauma, its multifaceted manifestations, and the mind's intricate defensive responses. I will expose the physical, mental, and emotional repercussions of trauma, unearthing the complex relationship between trauma and various health risks.

I will take you on a journey through my personal experiences and struggles, unmasking my fight with repressed memories, the roller coaster of diagnoses, and the path towards self-healing. My narrative is not only a testament to survival but an open letter for those who are facing similar battles.

A significant portion of this book is dedicated to the crucial role of mindset in trauma processing and healing. We'll dive into the pivotal factors that shape our mindset, from personal traumas to cultural programming and even the influence of DNA. With this knowledge, you'll be equipped to maintain a heightened sense of self-awareness and harness the power of your thoughts to alter your reality.

Furthermore, this book provides a detailed exploration of how to confront trauma head-on. The readers are promised an empowering narrative on the necessity of facing, understanding, and learning from our traumas. We will delve into the importance of boundary-setting, recognizing non-serving behaviors, and emphasizing the need for personal growth.

In essence, this book is not merely a narration of my experiences; it is a comprehensive guide promising you the tools to confront your own past, decipher your reactions, and pave the way towards a healthier future.

My journey will serve as a roadmap for you to embark on your journey towards self-discovery, healing, and personal development. It is a promise of transformation, resilience, and hope.

CHAPTER 2: UNRAVELING THE IMPACT OF ABUSE: A DEEP DIVE INTO MENTAL, EMOTIONAL, PHYSICAL, AND FINANCIAL MANIPULATION

Section I: Understanding The Different Types Of Abuse

Abuse, in its various forms, is a pervasive issue with profound effects on an individual's psychological well-being and life trajectory. While it can manifest in different ways, abuse always involves a pattern of behavior used to gain and maintain power and control over another person. The four primary forms we'll discuss in this chapter are mental, emotional, physical, and financial abuse.

Mental abuse, also known as psychological abuse, involves behaviors that affect a person's mind, leading them to feel isolated, fearful, or devalued. This form of abuse can include manipulation, gaslighting, and consistent criticism aimed at eroding an individual's confidence and self-esteem.

Emotional abuse, while closely related to mental abuse, is characterized by tactics aimed at damaging a person's emotional health and well-being. Emotional abusers often belittle, humiliate, and invalidate their victims' feelings, leading to chronic self-doubt, low self-esteem, and feelings of worthlessness.

Physical abuse involves intentional acts of violence or physical harm. These acts can range from hitting, slapping, and punching to more severe forms of violence. The physical scars can heal over time, but the emotional trauma left behind can persist for much longer.

Financial abuse involves controlling a person's ability to acquire, use, or maintain financial resources. This can include preventing someone from working, controlling their access to money, or making significant financial decisions without their consent. This form of abuse can lead to financial dependency, leaving the victim feeling trapped in their situation.

Section II: The Dire Effects of Abuse on the Psyche

Abuse, in any form, can have a severe and lasting impact on an individual's psyche. Victims often experience a wide range of mental health issues, including depression, anxiety, post-traumatic stress disorder (PTSD), and suicidal ideation.

These psychological effects can significantly interfere with the victim's daily life. They may struggle with self-worth, experience difficulties in forming healthy relationships, face challenges in their career progression, and even struggle with physical health problems caused by chronic stress and anxiety.

Section III: The Long-lasting Effects of Abuse

The effects of abuse often persist long after the abusive situation has ended. Survivors may grapple with feelings of fear, guilt, and shame, and their past experiences can impact their future relationships and interactions. Trust issues, intimacy problems, and self-esteem struggles are common among survivors of abuse.

Moreover, survivors of abuse are at a higher risk of developing various physical and mental health conditions, including chronic pain, insomnia, substance abuse disorders, and severe mental health conditions like depression and PTSD. They may also face financial difficulties, particularly in cases of financial abuse, as they strive to regain their independence and stability.

Section IV: Conclusion - The Urgency of Addressing Abuse Understanding the dire effects of abuse on the psyche underscores the critical need for early intervention, support, and recovery resources. While the journey to recovery may be challenging, it is indeed possible with the right support, resources, and resilience.

The next and final chapter will explore the healing process after experiencing abuse, focusing on the importance of professional help, self-care strategies, and supportive relationships. Furthermore, it will highlight the significance of resilience, its role in trauma recovery, and personal growth. The emphasis will be on embracing hope and forging a path towards healing, underscoring that the impacts of abuse do not have to define one's life permanently.

CHAPTER 3 – ANCESTRAL/ CULTURAL TRAUMA

Section I: Defining Ancestral/Cultural Trauma

Ancestral or cultural trauma refers to the collective emotional and psychological wounds suffered by a group of people across generations. This can include the residual effects of large-scale traumatic events that happened to previous generations, which impact the present generation in ways that may not be immediately apparent. This form of trauma is embedded in our collective memory, passed down through learned behaviors, implicit values, and shared emotional vulnerabilities.

Section II: The Influence of Culture and Ancestry

Our cultural heritage and ancestral lineage significantly influence our perspectives, behaviors, and attitudes. These elements shape our perception of the world, determining our role within our community and broader society. Are we givers or takers? Strivers or thrivers? These identities are largely influenced by the cultural values and ancestral lessons ingrained in us from a young age.

Cultural beliefs, traditions, and societal norms are embedded in our psyche from birth. They nourish our development and mold our personalities, impacting our outlook towards life and our sense of self. This ancestral and cultural upbringing sets the stage for our future successes, challenges, and how we navigate through life.

Section III: The Choice in Ancestral Lessons

Despite the considerable influence of our cultural and ancestral lineage, it's crucial to understand that these teachings or lessons are, ultimately, a choice. While our families and societies pass on certain values and beliefs, as individuals, we possess the autonomy to choose whether these ideas align with our personal values and life goals.

Understanding this provides an avenue for change, for breaking harmful cycles and patterns that have persisted through generations. We have the power to evaluate, question, and alter the beliefs and practices passed down to us, creating a new path that's in line with our personal growth and development.

Section IV: Breaking the Cycle

Breaking generational cycles requires self-awareness, understanding, and the courage to challenge deeply ingrained norms. It involves identifying the negative patterns in our families or culture, understanding their origins, and their impact on our current behaviors and beliefs. It's about acknowledging these harmful patterns and making a conscious decision to change.

Breaking the cycle involves seeking therapeutic interventions, educating oneself, and creating supportive networks. It's about establishing new, healthier patterns that foster growth, prosperity, and emotional well-being, not just for us but for future generations.

Suzanna Fraire

Section V: Personal Experience with Ancestral/Cultural Trauma

My personal experiences with ancestral and cultural trauma are a bit complex. My mother was a Japanese American military child raised in an era of segregation. Raised in an abusive, violent household was a victim of rape by a classmate in high school. Her narcissistic father then publicly killed the man, forcing my mother to testify against her own father and reliving her rape in open court. The inability to process these events, she fell for the first guy and got pregnant just to escape. Falling into the possession of a man who then proceeded to abuse her for several years physically, mentally, emotionally, and sexually. I share this story because I've known this story my whole life. I remember being younger than 10 years old and my mom pouring her heart out to me. The burden at that point became mine. I was a child dealing with adult things. I was obviously not qualified to address or even have knowledge of these issues. How it came back to me was, throughout my life, I would be subjected to similar experiences, not knowing how to navigate through them in a healthy manner. This is an extreme example of Ancestral Trauma. But it was in acknowledging my role and responsibilities in each cycle of trauma that ensued that I was able to change the narrative for my children. They did not endure the extent of abuse that she nor I endured. It was the choice that I made to not let those circumstances befall my children that broke those cycles. However, the choices I made were not always the greatest. Because I didn't have the coping skills I have today, I dumped on them different types of traumas, such as mental illness and addiction, which ultimately led to my suicide attempt.

If I had known then what I know now, the dynamics would be different.

My biological father disappeared for the most part prior to my birth. On the day I was born, he showed up, emptied out my mom's wallet and never looked back. This was after he ordered the doctors to perform a tubal ligation on her without her consent. The handful of memories I have of him and his family are riddled with physical, mental, emotional, and financial abuse.

How my cultural upbringing shaped my beliefs, behaviors, and perceptions and how I navigated the process of recognizing and breaking

Conversation With Myself
Managing the Madness of my Mind

free from harmful generational patterns. This is where my real dad comes into the picture. He met my mom when she was five months pregnant with me. For him, it was love at first sight. With him, he brought family, culture, customs, and structure to a woman fighting to pick up the pieces. He is patient, kind, giving, and nurturing. Loving her and supporting her until her dying day. He continues to shower me and my brother with unconditional love and support while still guiding us on a better path.

My dad is from Mexico and brought the traditions of old ways into our home. He was strict and overprotective and brought balance into our lives.

He gave us a family that is loving and accepting, loyal and true despite our faults. We are always united, even when we are not. We have each other's backs. It is in those traditions that I tried to raise my children. As life went on, it was in my ability to unconsciously choose to take the best and run with it that helped me survive. It was in those moments of female suppression that prove traumas arise out of the best of intentions. I was raised to be inferior to men. I was domesticated like an animal bred to be the docile wife and dutiful mother. I forwent my dreams of going to college to be a lawyer because I felt I had to live the path chosen for me. This created codependency issues and a lack of identity and self-worth. And it was because of this I wanted to raise my children in their own identities. I guess it worked for the most part, and they don't completely hate me. But the beauty is they have always known, whether consciously or unconsciously, that they can choose to take the best parts of me and release all the things that don't fit their narrative.

Section VI: The Power of Healing Ancestral/Cultural Trauma

Healing ancestral or cultural trauma involves rewriting our narrative and creating a new story that focuses on resilience, empowerment, and personal growth. It involves unlearning harmful behaviors and beliefs and replacing them with healthier alternatives.

Healing is a journey that requires courage, persistence, and patience. It's about acknowledging our past, understanding its impact on our present, and working towards a future that aligns with our true selves.

In the end, healing ancestral and cultural trauma gives us the power to redefine our identities, rewrite our stories, and reshape our destinies. It allows us to create a healthier and more empowering legacy for future generations.

CHAPTER 4 - SOCIETAL TRAUMA AND ITS IMPACTS

Section I: Understanding Societal Trauma

Societal trauma, much like personal trauma, has lasting and far-reaching effects. However, it differs in that it is experienced collectively. It stems from broad-scale events that impact a significant proportion of society, such as wars, genocides, terrorist attacks, pandemics, or social injustice, which can lead to shared trauma. In this chapter, we will delve into societal trauma, its effects, and how we, as individuals and societies, can navigate through it.

Section II: The Effects of Societal Trauma

Societal trauma can permeate every facet of life, affecting our mental, emotional, and physical well-being. It can lead to feelings of fear, anger, helplessness, and disillusionment. It can also cause more profound psychological effects like post-traumatic stress disorder (PTSD), anxiety, and depression. The most insidious aspect of societal trauma is its tendency to linger, leading to a state of chronic stress that impacts not only individuals but communities and societies as a whole.

Section III: Navigating Societal Trauma

Navigating societal trauma requires a collective response. As a society, we must acknowledge the traumatic event, understand its impact, and actively work towards healing and growth. This involves education, open dialogues, and sometimes seeking professional help, like therapy or counseling.

Remember, there is no single "right" way to navigate societal trauma - it is a personal journey that will differ for everyone.

Section IV: Personal Experience with Societal Trauma

My experience with societal trauma occurred amidst the political and societal upheaval in my country. Witnessing violence, unrest, and widespread fear had profound effects on me. It evoked feelings of anxiety and despair, but it also strengthened my resolve to work towards a more peaceful society. I'll share more about my experiences and the steps I took towards healing and resilience. These are my views and beliefs that align with me. This is in no way an attempt to inflict my beliefs on others.

Having grown up in a misogynist culture, it was hard for me to express my identity. And growing up in a society where every day my rights as a natural-born woman are being taken away is damning. In some states, we don't even have a right to our own bodies and the choices we make for the sake of our own well-being. Society is deciding what we, as humans in general, can do with our bodies. They deny us the basic benefits that are rewarded to those who are complaining. During the pandemic, the government enforced the stay-at-home order, imprisoning us in our own homes forcing those to find remote work or become unemployed, imposed the no vaccine, no work rule, leaving people with the options of either compromising their beliefs or feeding their families, they decreased supply and increased demand for basic human necessities such as food allowing companies to reduce their overall costs and increase their bottom line by reducing production and increasing prices. Big Pharma is creating cures for illness, only to be plagued by the side effects leading to a vicious cycle of addiction and reliance. Religions telling me that God will only love me if I follow a specific set of rules. That I will burn in hell if I choose to love a person of the same sex. Telling me I'm wrong if I choose to have an abortion, change my sex or if I identify as someone I wasn't born in this world to be. Why is it ok that society tells me what is right or wrong in my own being? Why does society get to impose these limitations? These are the conversations that clutter my mind.

Section V: The Role of Mindset and Coping Mechanisms

The mindset plays a critical role in how we cope with societal trauma. Having a positive, resilient mindset can help us navigate through tough times. It's also crucial to have healthy coping mechanisms, such as self-care routines, mindfulness practices, and supportive relationships. In this section, we'll explore different strategies to cultivate a resilient mindset and healthy coping mechanisms.

The first thing I did was eliminate external jargon that was influencing my thought process. I shut off the news; I removed myself from situations and people that didn't align with my beliefs and didn't support the need for growth and change. I imposed boundaries that empowered me to be who I am without self-judgment or reprimand. I focused on the things that brought positive feedback and outcomes in my life. I also focused on the things that are within my control to change. I realize that I cannot change the society as a whole. I can only change what is within me.

Section VI: The Power of Unity in Healing Societal Trauma

Healing from societal trauma is a collective effort. It involves coming together as a community, recognizing our shared experiences, and supporting each other in the healing process. It's in this unity that we find strength and resilience. Together, we can turn our traumatic experiences into a catalyst for positive societal change. It is imperative that we surround ourselves with like-minded people who are focused on change as a whole.

In the following chapters, we'll delve deeper into various types of trauma response tools and their effects, as well as the strategies for healing and growth. But remember, it's a journey, and every step you take towards understanding and healing is a step towards a better future for yourself and those around you.

CHAPTER 5 - DNA, HEREDITARY ILLNESS, AND TRAUMA: AN UNSEEN CONNECTION

Section I: The Genetics of Trauma

Genetics plays a significant role in how we understand trauma. Recent scientific studies have shown that the impact of traumatic events can be passed down through generations via our DNA, a concept known as epigenetic inheritance. In this section, we'll explore the intriguing and complex relationship between our genes and trauma, revealing how our ancestral experiences shape our responses to distressing events.

Section II: Understanding Hereditary Illness

Hereditary illnesses are conditions that can be passed from generation to generation through our genetic material. These illnesses, which range from physical conditions like heart disease or diabetes to mental health conditions like depression or schizophrenia, have a profound impact on the lives of those who inherit them. Living with a hereditary illness often creates its own set of challenges and traumas, affecting both the individual and their family members.

Section III: The Intersection of Hereditary Illness and Trauma

Hereditary illnesses can compound the effects of trauma in several ways. For one, they can make individuals more susceptible to the impacts of traumatic events due to their inherent health challenges. Moreover, the emotional toll of living with a chronic illness can heighten feelings of fear, anxiety, and vulnerability, enhancing the impact of any subsequent traumatic events. In this section, we'll delve into these connections in more depth, shedding light on the intricate interplay of genetics, health, and trauma.

Section IV: Personal Experiences with Hereditary Illness and Trauma

I have personal experience with hereditary illness and the trauma it can cause. In my family, there is a history of clinical depression, bipolar disorder, cancer, heart disease, diabetes, obesity and more. These genetic predispositions have affected several generations and shaped the lives of my family members in profound ways. I share my story in this section, hoping to provide insight and foster understanding about the very real impacts of hereditary illness and trauma.

It wasn't easy caring for my mother towards the end of her life. She was in denial about being predisposed to these hereditary diseases and even more so about having them. She was very non-compliant with her treatment plans and refused help along the way.

It was up to me to acknowledge that these illnesses could become my story and change the narrative. I had to look at her lifestyle choices and those of the family, past and present. I had to create a plan to stop the cycle so my children and grandchildren could lead healthy, happy, and productive lives.

Section V: Coping Strategies for Hereditary Illness and Trauma

Living with a hereditary illness can be challenging, but there are ways to cope with these challenges and mitigate the associated trauma. This section will discuss various coping strategies, from seeking professional help like counseling and therapy to cultivating a supportive network of friends and family. We'll also look at how self-care practices, mindfulness, and resilience can support individuals in managing the dual burden of hereditary illness and trauma.

Managing a hereditary illness or chronic illness is a lifestyle. We must learn to nourish our bodies with the nutrients they need for optimal health. We must use the resources available to us to maximize our longevity. It is important to incorporate various methods of healing to reach optimal health, both mentally and physically. Understanding that science and Big Pharma are just one method of managing health. We must also incorporate our own bodies' capacity to self-regulate. Through meditation and holistic medicine, we are able to achieve a healthy lifestyle as well.

Section VI: The Power of Knowledge and Awareness

Understanding the influence of our genes on our health and emotional responses is empowering. It enables us to take proactive steps towards managing our health and mental well-being. Knowledge about our genetic predispositions can help us navigate life with more consciousness and compassion, not just for ourselves but for those around us as well.

In the upcoming chapters, we'll explore more about trauma responses and delve into various strategies for healing and growth. Remember, everyone's journey is unique, and every step taken towards understanding and healing is a stride towards a healthier, more resilient future.

CHAPTER 6 - MENTAL BLOCKS AND THE IMPACT OF A CLOSED MIND: BARRIERS TO GROWTH

Section I: Understanding Mental Blocks

Mental blocks are psychological obstacles that hinder our ability to think, act, and progress. These may stem from a variety of factors, including past trauma, stress, anxiety, fear of failure, or deeply ingrained belief systems. Mental blocks can significantly impact our productivity, creativity, emotional health, and overall personal growth. In this section, we will delve deeper into the nature of mental blocks and their potential sources.

Section II: The Impact of a Closed Mind

A closed mind is a mental state characterized by an unwillingness to consider new ideas, perspectives, or experiences. While it might offer the comfort of familiarity, a closed mind limits personal growth, fosters intolerance, and impedes problem-solving abilities. It can lead to stagnation, both on a personal and societal level, as it hinders our capacity to learn, adapt, and evolve. In this section, we will explore the far-reaching implications of having a closed mind.

It is my belief that having a closed mind limits our capacity to reach our full potential. By not exploring all available resources and options, we are bound to continue to live unhealthy, unhappy lives. And when we are in such a negative state, we are not allowing our body's natural process. There are times when medications are necessary. They are created to improve where the body lacks, such as diabetes medication, to regulate the production of insulin in our body. But we must constantly ask ourselves, why is our body out of sync? What can I do in addition to the medications available? And most importantly, take the steps needed to improve our current state.

Section III: The Intersection of Mental Blocks and Closed Mind

Mental blocks and a closed mind often go hand in hand. The fear, anxiety, or inflexibility that results in mental blocks can also lead to a closed mindset. Conversely, a closed mind can perpetuate mental blocks by discouraging us from seeking new ways to overcome our challenges. Together, they form a vicious cycle that can be hard to break. Here, we will discuss how these two factors intersect and the collective impact they can have on our lives.

Section IV: Personal Experiences with Mental Blocks and a Closed Mind

In this section, I will share my own experiences grappling with mental blocks and maintaining a closed mind. As a survivor of various forms of trauma, I've had to confront significant mental barriers and grapple with the damaging effects of a closed mind. By sharing my experiences, I hope to offer a candid look into the realities of these struggles and highlight the importance of seeking growth and openness.

Having a long list of diagnoses, physical and mental, I was consuming 22 pills a day. They included therapies for antipsychotics to manage my bipolar disorder, borderline personality disorder, depression, anxiety, and manic behavior. I was also taking a cocktail of vitamins for malnutrition and chronic fatigue issues due to having had a gastric bypass almost 20 years ago to overcome obesity. And then came the narcotics to relieve the pain from fibromyalgia and migraines. I was a ticking time bomb. I couldn't live in that box anymore. I needed a better quality of life, not just for myself but for my family as well. I saw firsthand how this contributed to the failure of my marriage. I saw the effects it was having on my children and others around me. This was no longer acceptable to me.

Section V: Strategies for Overcoming Mental Blocks and Opening Your Mind

Despite the challenges posed by mental blocks and a closed mind, there are numerous strategies that can help us overcome these barriers. These include cognitive techniques, mindfulness practices, therapy, and fostering an attitude of curiosity and openness. This section will provide practical advice on how to navigate mental blocks and cultivate an open mind.

I was desperate for change. My overdose in 2016, just after my mom died, was my turning point. The look in my son's eyes when he found me unconscious on my bed is forever seared in my brain. The pain and suffering they endured watching me lose myself. I can only imagine how helpless, angry, and sad they felt, wondering why their love wasn't enough to make me happy. Living in fear day after day that I'd be gone forever. Losing their faith and trust has been my greatest regret in life. But it is in that I choose to live each day in hopes of regaining it back. And although I may never completely have it, I will never stop trying. They inspire me every moment of every day, and it is in healing myself and changing the future that I know heals the traumas of their past. Because, what I know for sure, is that they are better than me, and they will never make their children suffer the way they did.

Section VI: The Power of an Open Mind and Overcoming Mental Blocks

Overcoming mental blocks and cultivating an open mind are empowering steps towards personal growth and fulfillment. They enhance our capacity to learn, adapt, and flourish, even in the face of adversity. They also encourage empathy, understanding, and unity on a societal level. In this concluding section, we'll reflect on the power of adopting an open mindset and overcoming mental blocks.

In the last chapter, we will continue to explore the impact of trauma on various aspects of our lives, along with the tools and strategies that can aid in healing and growth. Remember, every step taken towards understanding and healing is a stride towards a more resilient future.

CHAPTER 7

Cognitive-Behavioral Therapy (CBT), Dialectical Behavioral Therapy (DBT), Neuro-Linguistic Programming (NLP), Trans Magnetic Stimulation (TMS) and Meditation: Tools for Healing and Growth

Section I: Understanding Cognitive-Behavioral Therapy (CBT)

Cognitive-Behavioral Therapy (CBT) is a form of psychotherapy that addresses maladaptive thought patterns in order to change negative behaviors and emotions. CBT is predicated on the belief that our thoughts, not external factors, dictate our feelings and behaviors. This therapy helps individuals identify, challenge, and replace cognitive distortions and improve coping strategies.

Section II: The Role of Dialectical Behavioral Therapy (DBT)

Dialectical Behavioral Therapy (DBT) is another form of cognitive-behavioral therapy. It was originally developed to treat borderline personality disorder but is now widely used for a variety of mental health conditions. DBT focuses on acceptance and change, helping individuals to tolerate distress, regulate emotions, be more mindful, and improve interpersonal effectiveness.

Section III: The Power of Neuro-Linguistic Programming (NLP)

Neuro-Linguistic Programming (NLP) is a psychological approach that involves analyzing strategies used by successful individuals and applying them to reach personal goals. NLP examines patterns of behavior and provides techniques to facilitate change. It is used for self-development and for improving interpersonal communication.

Section IV: Transcranial Magnetic Stimulation: A Contemporary Approach

Transcranial Magnetic Stimulation (TMS) is an innovative, non-invasive treatment method used primarily for treating major depressive disorder and various other mental health conditions. This technique harnesses the power of magnetic fields to stimulate nerve cells in the brain, particularly those regions linked to mood control and depression.

The process involves placing an electromagnetic coil against the patient's scalp near the forehead. The electromagnet delivers a painless magnetic pulse that stimulates nerve cells in the region of the brain involved in mood regulation and depression. This technique is usually employed when other standard treatments, such as medication or psychotherapy, have proven ineffective.

In my personal experience, TMS was another critical tool that significantly aided in my mental health recovery journey. I found it particularly useful in managing my depression symptoms when traditional therapeutic approaches fell short. The treatment sessions, which lasted for a few weeks, became an integral part of my overall mental health management plan.

Post-treatment, I experienced noticeable improvements in my mood, cognitive function, and overall emotional well-being. The decrease in the intensity of depressive symptoms, coupled with improved emotional regulation, was a significant turning point in my mental health journey.

It's important to note that while TMS has been beneficial to many people like me, its effectiveness can vary between individuals. As with any treatment, it should be discussed thoroughly with a healthcare provider to determine its suitability based on your personal medical history and current health status.

Ultimately, TMS serves as an exemplar of the exciting advances in mental health treatment. By harnessing the power of technology and deepening our understanding of the brain, we continue to push the boundaries of what's possible in mental health recovery.

Section V: The Benefits of Meditation

Meditation is an ancient practice that involves focusing the mind and achieving a mentally clear and emotionally calm state. Regular meditation has been shown to reduce stress, increase focus, improve mental clarity, enhance emotional well-being, and promote overall health. The beauty of meditation lies in its simplicity and versatility, making it a tool that anyone, regardless of age or experience, can incorporate into their routine.

Section VI: Personal Experiences with CBT, DBT, NLP, TMS, and Meditation

In this section, I'll share my experiences with each of these therapeutic approaches. From working through cognitive distortions with CBT, learning to manage emotional intensity with DBT, and enhancing self-awareness with NLP, to finding inner peace through meditation, my journey has been transformative.

In my struggle to manage numerous mental health diagnoses and chronic pain, I found myself relying heavily on pharmaceutical interventions.

While they did provide some relief, I felt that they were merely a band-aid solution. They didn't address the root cause of my pain. It was at this point that I turned to alternative therapeutic approaches—CBT, DBT, NLP, TMS and Meditation.

Section VII: The Power of CBT, DBT, NLP, TMS, and Meditation

The potential of these therapeutic techniques becomes particularly salient through the lens of personal experiences. The combination of CBT, DBT, NLP, TMS, and meditation provided me with a broader perspective on my struggles, granting me more control over my reactions and facilitating a journey towards a healthier and more fulfilling life.

Cognitive-Behavioral Therapy (CBT) helped me recognize and challenge my negative thought patterns. By questioning these ingrained beliefs and assumptions, I was able to replace them with more positive and productive thoughts. This shift in mindset was a significant catalyst for change, enabling me to handle stress and emotional turbulence more effectively.

Dialectical Behavioral Therapy (DBT), on the other hand, equipped me with the skills to navigate emotional extremes. Through DBT, I learned how to tolerate distress without resorting to destructive coping mechanisms, manage intense emotions without getting overwhelmed, and communicate effectively in relationships. The impact of these skills cannot be overstated. They not only improved my emotional well-being but also enhanced the quality of my interpersonal relationships.

Neuro-Linguistic Programming (NLP) offered yet another layer of personal insight. It helped me recognize my behavioral patterns and how they were linked to my thoughts and feelings. By understanding these connections, I was able to make positive changes that affected my overall outlook and interactions with others. It was as though I had been handed the blueprint for my mental processes and could finally remodel it for the better.

Meditation, while often viewed as a standalone practice, became an essential element in my toolkit. It has provided a safe space for me to connect with myself and cultivate mindfulness - a skill that significantly benefits all other areas of my life. It brought about a sense of tranquility and balance, even in the midst of chaos.

The synergy of these therapies opened up a path of healing and personal growth that I never thought was possible. They didn't merely alleviate my symptoms but addressed the underlying issues that perpetuated my pain. By embracing these therapeutic strategies, I was able to transcend my past traumas and evolve into a more resilient, balanced, and self-aware individual.

It's worth mentioning, however, that while these therapies were instrumental in my healing process, they may not necessarily work for everyone in the same way. Everyone's journey is unique, and what works for one might not work for another. Nevertheless, these therapies offer a myriad of strategies that can be tailored to individual needs and circumstances, making them a valuable resource for anyone on the path of personal growth.

The power of these therapeutic techniques lies in their capacity to facilitate lasting change. They are not quick fixes but rather tools for deep-seated transformation. By adopting these strategies, we don't just learn to cope with our struggles - we learn to thrive despite them. Through this transformative journey, we move closer to a healthier, more resilient future.

CONCLUSION:

The Significance of Resilience in Trauma Recovery and Personal Growth

The journey of healing and growth is far from linear. It is fraught with challenges and setbacks that may often seem insurmountable. Yet, it is through navigating these hurdles that we begin to tap into our innate resilience. Resilience, in its essence, is the capacity to recover from difficulties and spring back into shape in the face of adversity. It is not about avoiding hardship but about learning how to adapt and persevere in its presence.

In the context of trauma recovery, resilience plays a critical role. Trauma can shatter our sense of safety, undermine our self-esteem, and leave us feeling broken. But through resilience, we can learn to process these painful experiences, rebuild our trust, and start to heal. It's resilience that enables us to look beyond our past traumas and envision a future where we are not defined by our wounds but by how we've risen from them.

Similarly, in the realm of personal growth, resilience equips us with the strength to persist on our path of self-discovery and self-improvement. As we traverse this path, we inevitably encounter roadblocks - failures, rejections, self-doubt, and fear. Resilience encourages us not to perceive these as terminal setbacks but as learning opportunities. It inspires us to confront our fears, learn from our failures, and continue to grow despite them.

Embracing the practices and therapies we've explored in this chapter, such as CBT, DBT, NLP, TMS, and meditation, can significantly contribute to nurturing our resilience. As we learn to manage our emotions, challenge our negative thought patterns, enhance our cognitive function, and cultivate mindfulness, we are, in fact, reinforcing our resilience. We are equipping ourselves with the skills and mindset necessary to navigate the inevitable ups and downs of life, thereby fostering our ability to bounce back from adversity.

In conclusion, the power of resilience in trauma recovery and personal growth is immense. It's the thread that holds our healing journey together, binding our pain, our growth, and our strength into a tapestry of transformation. Remember, it's not the absence of adversity that defines our journey but the resilience we embody in its face. As we continue on this path, let's celebrate our resilience and acknowledge the tremendous strength within us. The journey ahead may be challenging, but with resilience at our core, we are more than capable of facing whatever comes our way.

Here are some resources for various therapeutic approaches and mental health support:

- Cognitive-Behavioral Therapy (CBT)

The Association for Behavioral and Cognitive Therapies: www.abct.org
The Beck Institute for Cognitive Behavior Therapy: www.beckinstitute.org

- Dialectical Behavioral Therapy (DBT)

The Linehan Institute: www.linehaninstitute.org
DBT Self Help: www.dbtselfhelp.com

- Neuro-Linguistic Programming (NLP)

The NLP Center: www.nlpu.com
The NLP Academy: www.nlpacademy.co.uk

- Transcranial Magnetic Stimulation (TMS)

National Institute of Mental Health (NIMH): www.nimh.nih.gov
Mayo Clinic: www.mayoclinic.org

- Meditation

The Mindfulness App: www.mindfulnessapp.com
Headspace: www.headspace.com

- Mental Health Resources

National Suicide Prevention Lifeline: 1-800-273-TALK (1-800-273-8255) or 988 suicidepreventionlifeline.org
SAMHSA's National Helpline: 1-800-662-HELP (1-800-662-4357)
www.samhsa.gov
Crisis Text Line: Text "HELLO" to 741741 www.crisistextline.org

Conversation With Myself
Managing the Madness of my Mind

The Trevor Project (for LGBTQ+ youth): 1-866-488-7386 or text "START" to 678678 www.thetrevorproject.org

Please remember, in case of an emergency, always call your local emergency number immediately.

These resources are meant to provide general wellness and are not a substitute for professional help. Always consult with a healthcare provider for appropriate treatment and therapy options.

ABOUT THE AUTHOR

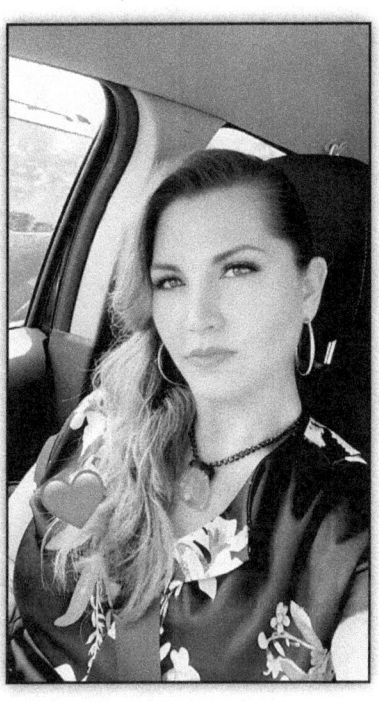

Suzanna Fraire was born and raised in the Bay Area, California. She is the mother of three magnificent boys and a grandmother. She has been diagnosed with bipolar disorder, borderline personality disorder, mania, anxiety, and depression. She has spent the last six years managing her madness through various techniques, beliefs, and practices, exploring the depths of her mind, and expanding it to its full potential.

www.ingramcontent.com/pod-product-compliance
Lightning Source LLC
Chambersburg PA
CBHW070338120526
44590CB00017B/2938